Fast Fat Burning Green Smoothie Recipes

Turn the Greens into Tasty Sips

Disclaimer

All Rights Reserved. Any content of this publication cannot be replicated or transmitted by any means or in any form including electronic, print, photocopying, recording, or scanning without written consent from the publication's author.

The author has tried to be an authentic source of the information provided in this report. However, the author does not oppose the additional information available over the internet. The objective of providing different Green Smoothie recipes is to enable readers to try these delicious and healthy recipes at home. The information included in this book cannot be compared with the preparation methods of such smoothies provided in other books. All readers can seek further help through additional sources of information.

Ignoring any of the guidelines or not following each step of the preparation method of green smoothies may not give you the exact result. Therefore, the author is not responsible for such negligence.

Table of Contents

The Introduction: What Is So Good About Green Smoothies? 5
Green Smoothie Recipes 6
    Green Apple Smoothie 6
    Green Smoothie with Tea, Kiwi, and Mango 7
    Sunrise Smoothie 9
    All-Green Smoothie 11
    Green Monster Smoothie 13
    Papaya Mint Smoothie 15
    Spinach-Mango Smoothie Recipe 17
    Spinach Smoothie with Pear and Celery 18
    Mixed-Berries Smoothie 19
    Spinach and Blueberry Smoothie 21
    Spinach and Tropical Fruit Smoothie 22
    Spinach-Kiwi Green Smoothie 23
    Spinach Smoothie with Watermelon and Strawberries 24
    Orange Smoothie with Spinach and Banana 25
    Spinach and Tomato Smoothie 26
    Green Limeade Smoothie 27
    Grapes Smoothie 29
    Kale Smoothie 30
    Avocado Smoothie 31
    Honeydew Melon Smoothie 32
    Ginger and Spinach Smoothie 33
    Green Coconut Smoothie with Spinach 34
    Green Apple and Cinnamon Smoothie 35
    Low-Fat Honey and Green Tea Smoothie 36
    Dandelion Green Smoothie 37
    Green Fruity Smoothie 38
    Mixed Greens Smoothie 40
    Collard Green Smoothie 41

Kiwi Smoothie with Berry and Collards 43
Fresh Collard Smoothie with Strawberries 44
Final Word 46

The Introduction: What Is So Good About Green Smoothies?

If you are new to adopt green smoothies to your lifestyle, it is important to mention here that a glass of green smoothie can be everything you need to begin your day with! With its unlimited health benefits, it gives you much more than that. A good taste and vitality is the perfect combination you can get from drinking a green smoothie.

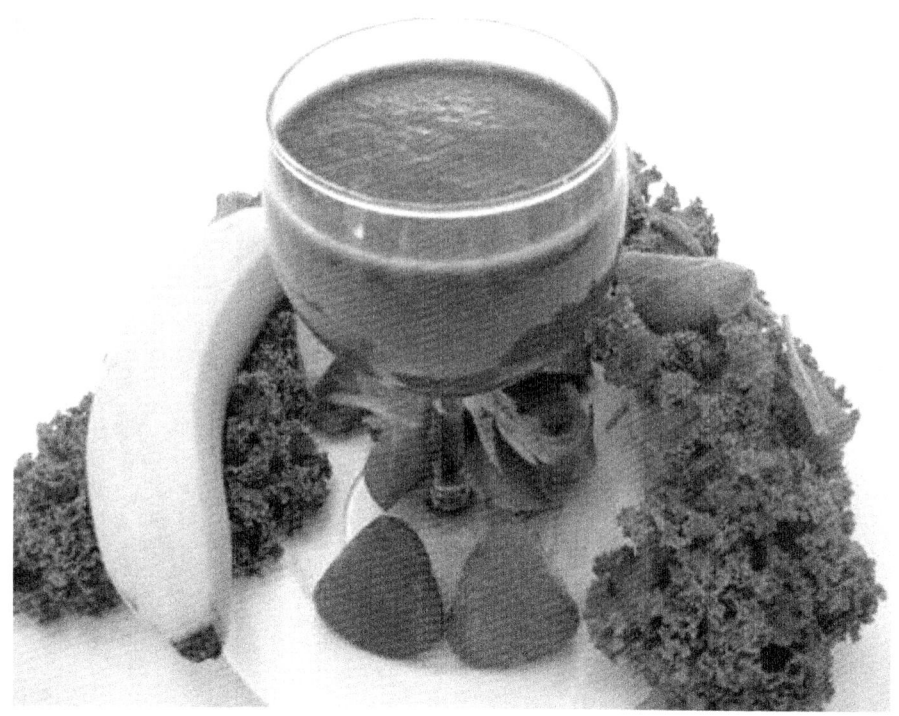

So, why not enjoy it with your friends and family? It is easy to prepare green smoothies at home. Green Smoothie recipes given in this book will help you throughout the process of preparing them the right way.

Green Smoothie Recipes

Green Apple Smoothie

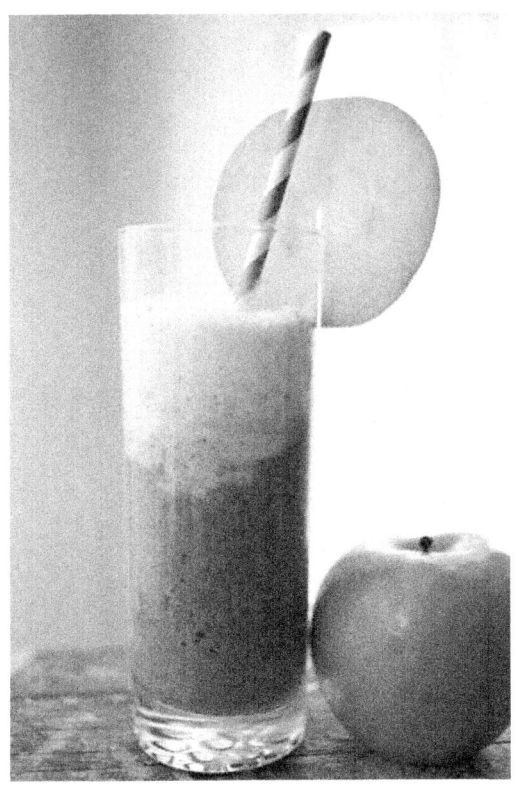

Ingredients

Banana: 1

Organic apple (cored): 1

Organic spinach (fresh): 2 cups

Flaxseeds: 2 teaspoons

Crushed ice: 1 ½ cups

Directions

Blend all the ingredients until they are smooth. Your refreshing drink is ready.

Green Smoothie with Tea, Kiwi, and Mango

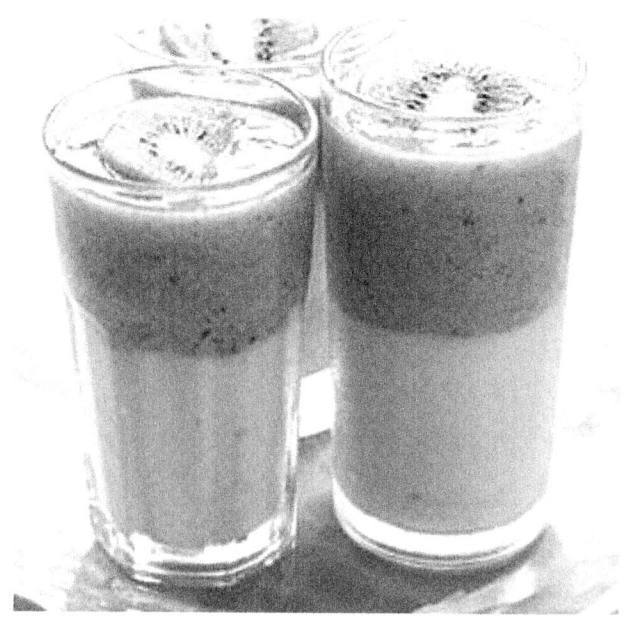

Ingredients

Mangos (frozen, diced): 2 ½ cups

Vanilla yogurt (fat-free, divided): ¾ cup

Honey (divided): ¼ cup

Water: 2 tablespoons

Lime peel (grated): ½ teaspoon

Ripe kiwifruit (peeled, cut in quarters): 3

Ice cubes: 2 cups

Baby spinach (packed): ½ cup

Green tea (bottled): 2 tablespoons

Kiwifruit slices: optional

Directions

1. Take a blender, and place mango, 2 tablespoons of honey, ½ cup of vanilla yogurt, 2 tablespoons of water, and lime peel in it. Process them until you get smooth mango mixture. Stir occasionally.

2. Now take 4 smoothie glasses, and divide the mango mixture in each of them. Place these glasses in the freezer.

3. Rinse the blender container. After this, place 2 tablespoons of honey, ¼ cup of yogurt, kiwifruit, baby spinach, green tea, and ice cubes in the blender. Process all these ingredients until they are smooth. Stir occasionally.

4. Now, take out the smoothie glasses from freezer. Gently spoon the second mixture onto the mango mixture in these glasses. Make sure that you create a neat horizontal line inside each glass.

5. Once this is done, you can garnish the smoothies with slices of kiwifruit. Also, if you want to combine flavors, simply stir to get a tastier flavor.

Sunrise Smoothie

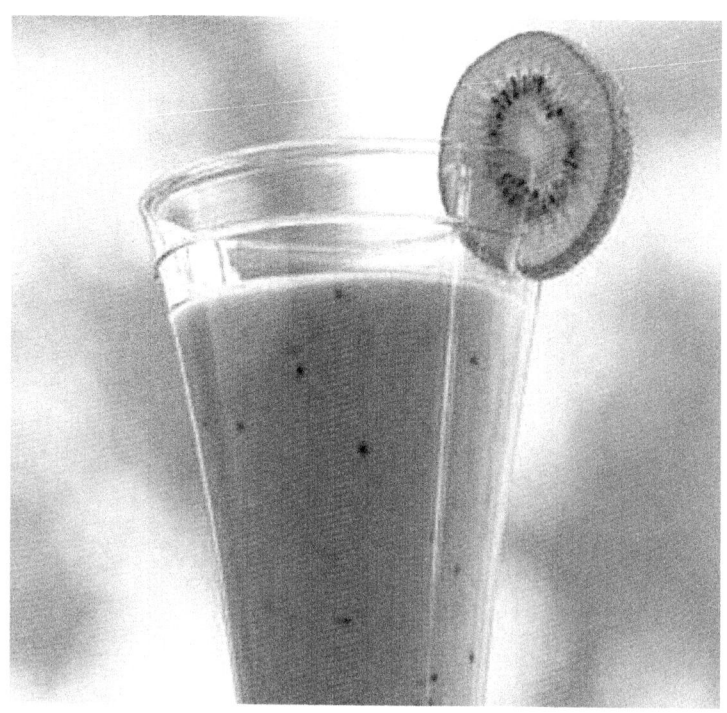

Ingredients

Kiwifruit (peeled and cubed): 4, i.e. ¾ pound

Ripe bananas (medium-sized, cut in 1-inch slices)

Green tea bags (fruit-flavored): 4

Boiled soy milk (low-fat): 1 ½ cups

Honey: 1 tablespoon

Directions

1. Take a large-sized zipped plastic bag, and place banana slices and cubed kiwifruit in it. Seal the bag and place it in freezer for about thirty minutes or till the fruits become almost firm.

2. Meanwhile, take a medium-sized bowl, and place tea bags in it. Pour boiling low-fat soy milk over these tea bags. Steep for three minutes.

3. Take a sieve and use it to strain this tea mixture into another bowl. Discard the used teabags. Now, stir in honey. Let it cool. The tea mixture is ready.

4. Now, combine bananas and kiwifruit in the same tea mixture. Place this mixture into a blender, and process it well till you get a smooth mixture. Sunrise smoothie is ready to be served.

All-Green Smoothie

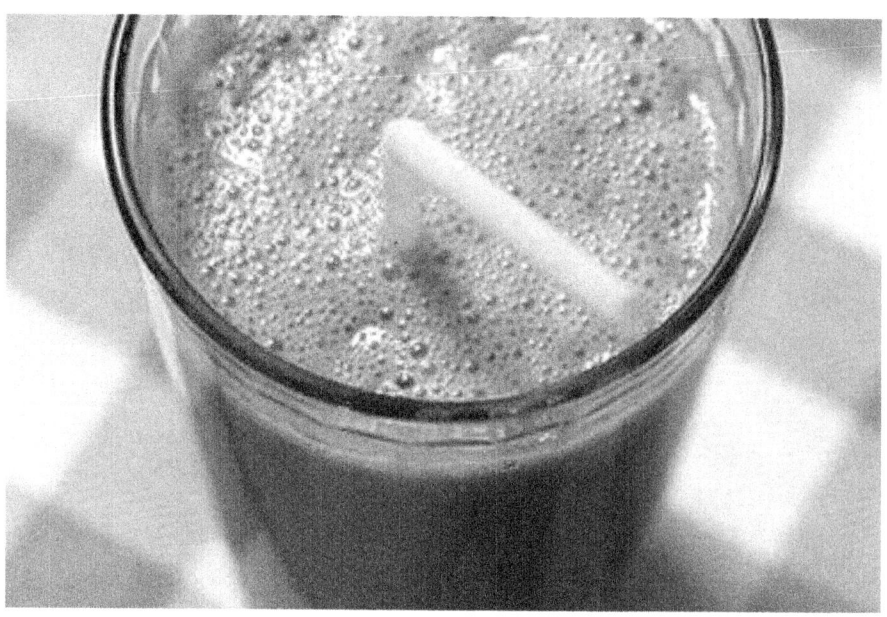

Ingredients

Water: ¼ cup

Pineapple juice: ½ cup

Green grapes: 1 ¾ cups

Ripe Bartlett pear (seeded, halved)

Avocado (pitted and peeled): ½ piece

Broccoli (coarsely chopped): ¼ cup

Spinach (washed): ½ cup

Ice cubes: ¼ cup

Directions

1. Take a blender, and pour all the ingredients into it. Switch it on slow speed at first. Wait for 3 to 4 seconds and increase the speed.

2. Blend for thirty-five to forty seconds or till you get a smooth mixture. All-Green Smoothie is ready to drink.

Note: You can add a bit of water into it if it is extra thick.

Green Monster Smoothie

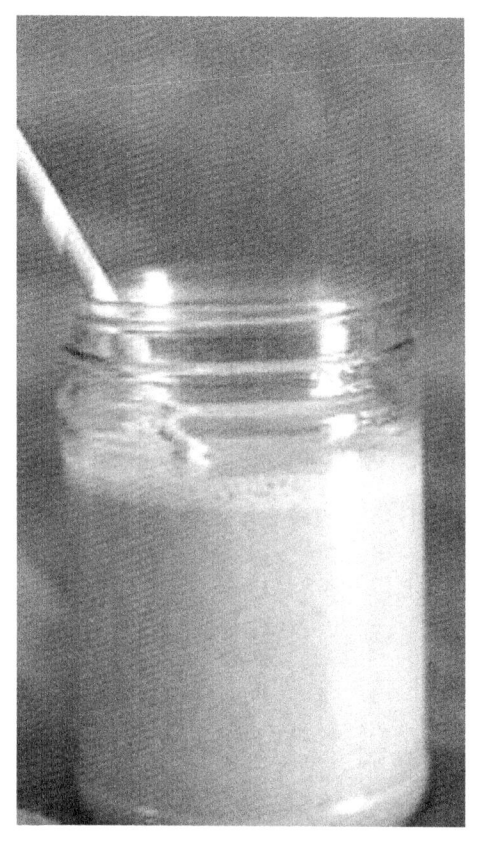

Ingredients

Banana (sliced and frozen): 1

Peanut butter: ½ tablespoons

Greek yogurt (low-fat): ½ cup

Honey: 1 tablespoon

Almond milk: 1 cup

Baby spinach: 4 cups

Directions

1. Rinse all the ingredients thoroughly.

2. Take a blender, and place them in it. Blend them until you get a smooth mixture. If you do not want highly thick smoothie, add a bit of water. Refrigerate it to enjoy the awesome taste of Green Monster Smoothie.

Papaya Mint Smoothie

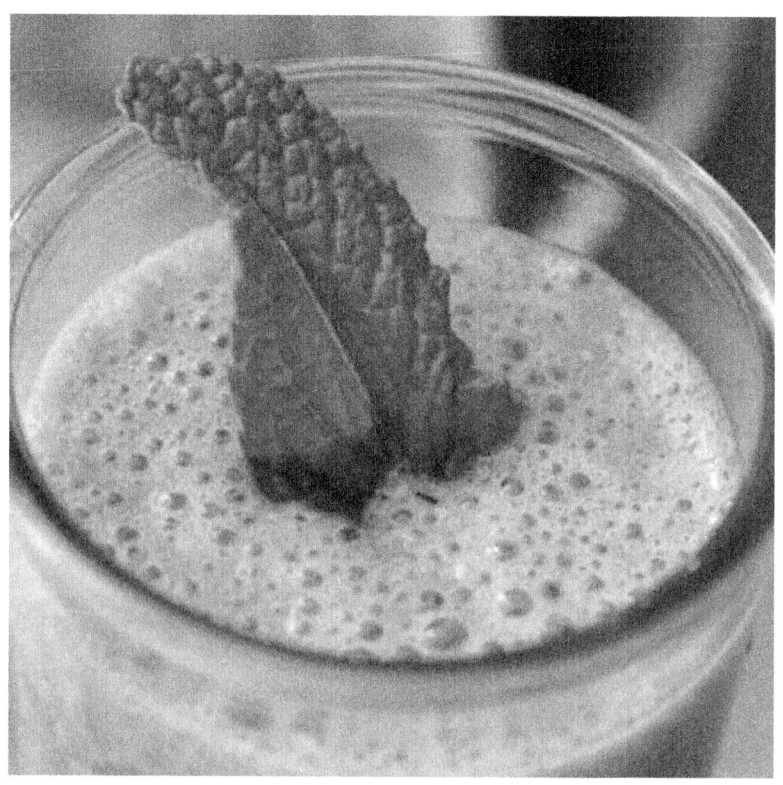

Ingredients

Papaya (cubed): 2 cups

Pear (cored): 1

Spinach (fresh or frozen): 3 cups

Mint leaves (fresh): 10

Goji berries (dried): 2 tablespoons

Filtered water: 8 oz

Directions

1. Take a blender, and place the soft fruits in it first. Start processing until they form a smooth mixture.

2. Now add other ingredients. Place the greens last. Now, blend these ingredients on high speed. This will take about 30 seconds. However, the blending duration depends on how quickly

you get a smooth mixture. So, when it is smooth enough, switch off the blender. Papaya mint smoothie is ready.

Note: A high-speed blender is required to prepare the Papaya Mint Smoothie. If you do not have one, then you can soften the goji berries by soaking them in water for about 10 minutes. After this, you can add them with other ingredients in your blender.

Spinach-Mango Smoothie Recipe

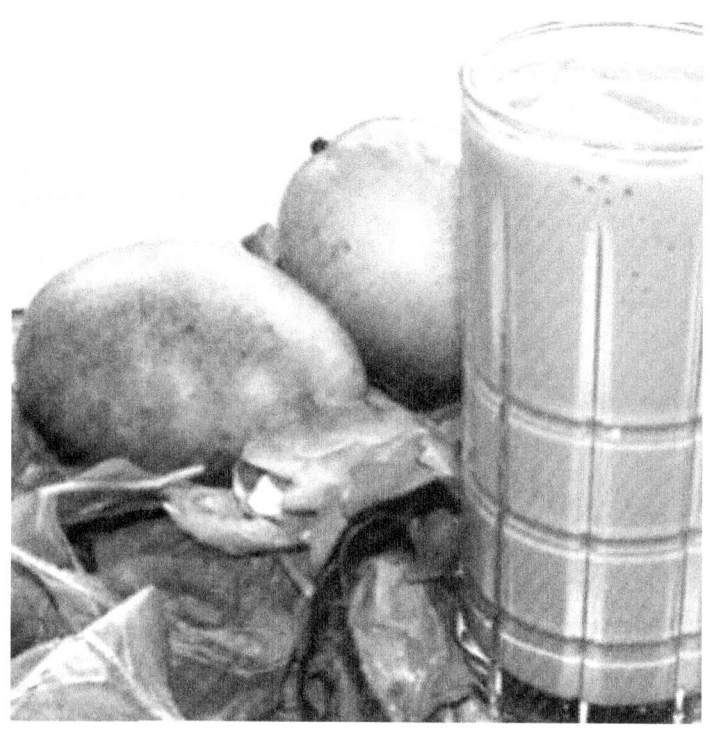

Ingredients

Ripe banana (large): 1

Mangoes: 1 cup (cut in small slices)

Strawberries: ½ cup

Spinach: 5 oz

Water: 1 ½ cups

Directions

Take a blender and put all the ingredients in it. Process the ingredients until they turn into a smooth mixture. Pour the smoothie into a tall glass. It is ready to drink.

Spinach Smoothie with Pear and Celery

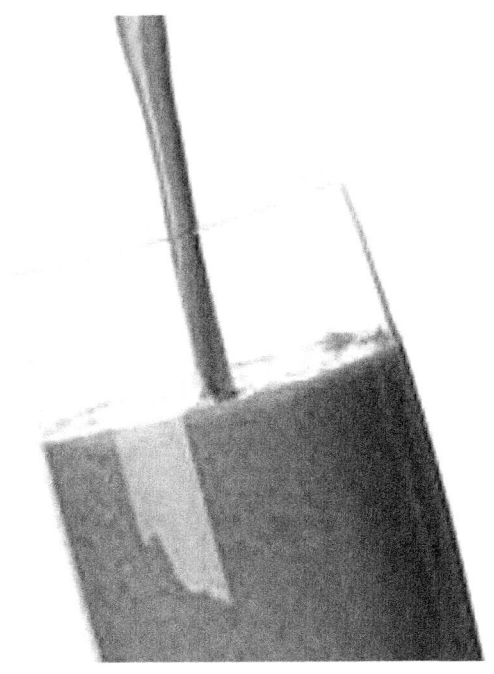

Ingredients

Pears: 2

Celery: 2 stalks

Spinach: 2 cups

Water: 1 ½ cup

Directions

Blend all the ingredients in a blender. Pour the green smoothie into glasses. Enjoy the taste of celery and pear.

Mixed-Berries Smoothie

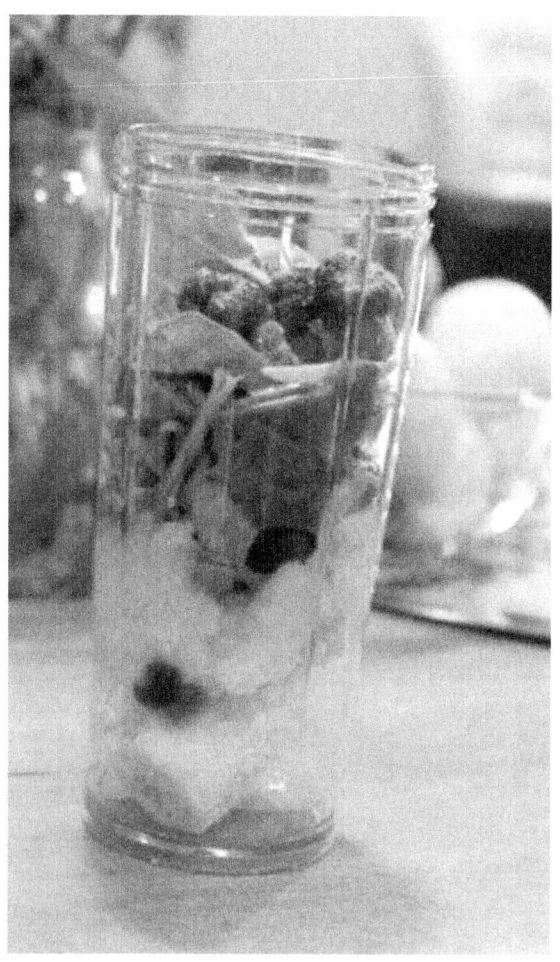

Ingredients

Fresh spinach: 2 to 4 cups

Strawberries (fresh/frozen): a handful

Blueberries (fresh/frozen): ½ cup

Blackberries (fresh/frozen): 1/4 cup

Raspberries (fresh/frozen): ¼ cup

Bananas (fresh/frozen): 2 cups

Water: 1 ½ cups

Directions

Blend all the ingredients in a blender. Process till you see them turning into a smooth and think liquid. If you are unable to get all the berries, you can use 1 cup of mixed froze berries while preparing this smoothie.

Spinach and Blueberry Smoothie

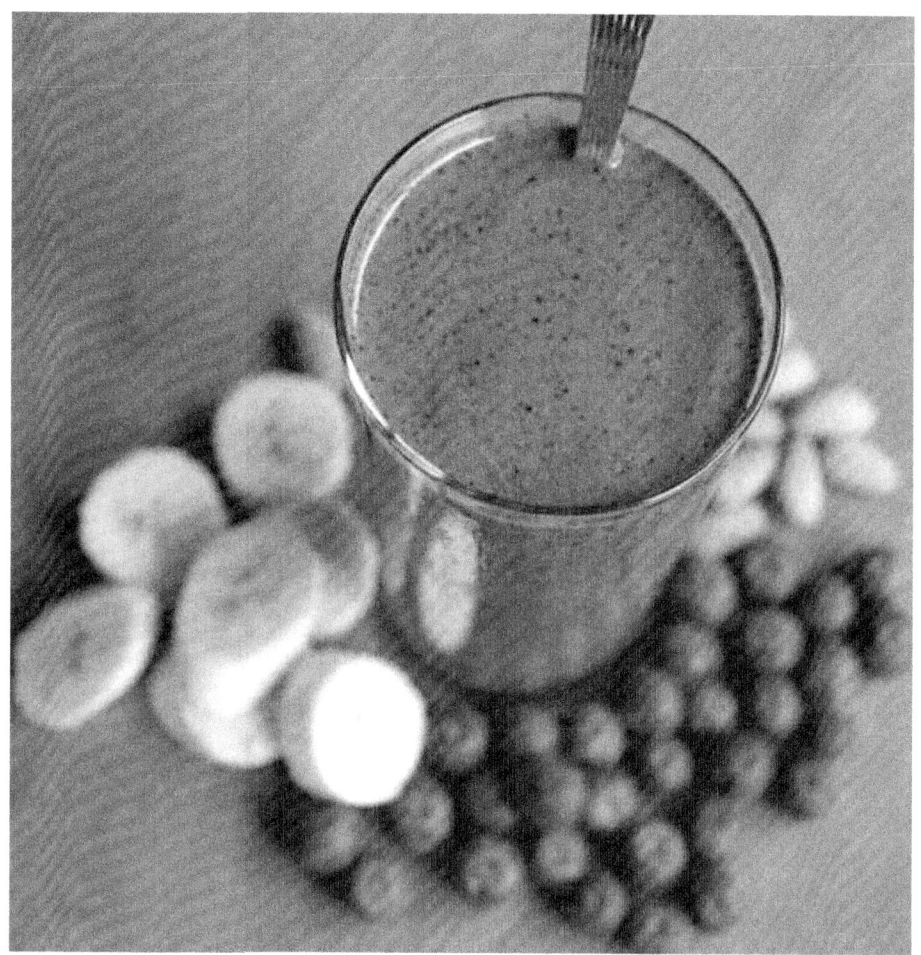

Ingredients

Ripe banana (large): 1

Frozen blueberries: 1 cup

Fresh spinach: 1 cup

Water: 1 ½ cups

Directions

Blend all the ingredients well. Spinach and blueberry smoothie is ready to drink. You can add less or more water into it, depending on the way you like it. If you prefer to make it less think, then add more water.

Spinach and Tropical Fruit Smoothie

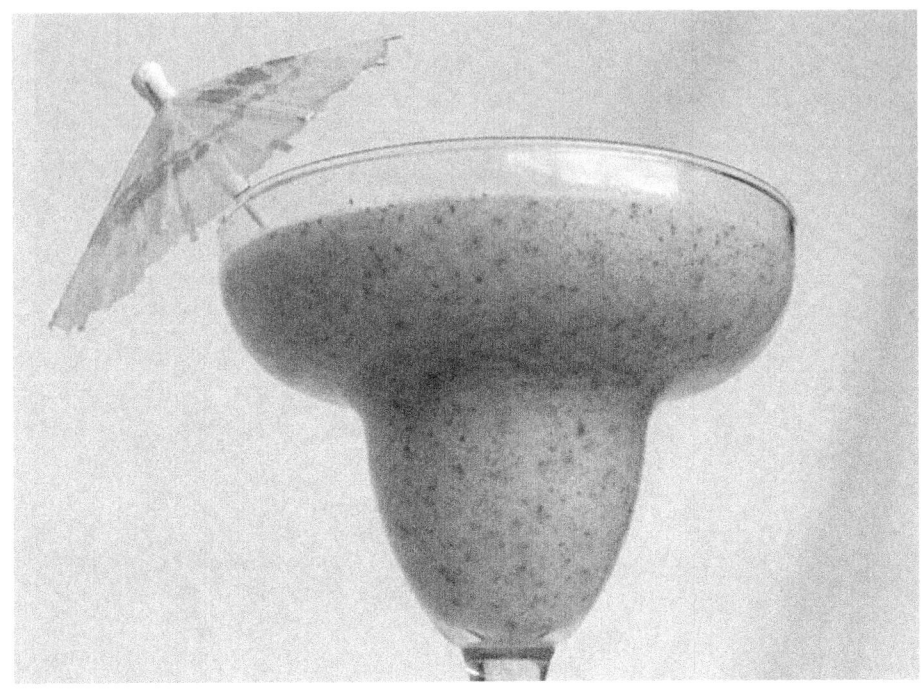

Ingredients

Ripe banana (large, peeled): 1

Avocado: ¼ cup

Fresh spinach: 6 oz

Pineapple (frozen or fresh): ½ cup

Mango (frozen or fresh): ½ cup

Grapes (frozen or fresh): ½ cup

Strawberries (frozen or fresh): ½ cup

Water: 1 ½ cup

Directions

Take a food processor or blender and pour all the ingredients in it. Process them until smooth. Add more water if desirable. Spinach and Tropical Fruit smoothie is ready to drink.

Spinach-Kiwi Green Smoothie

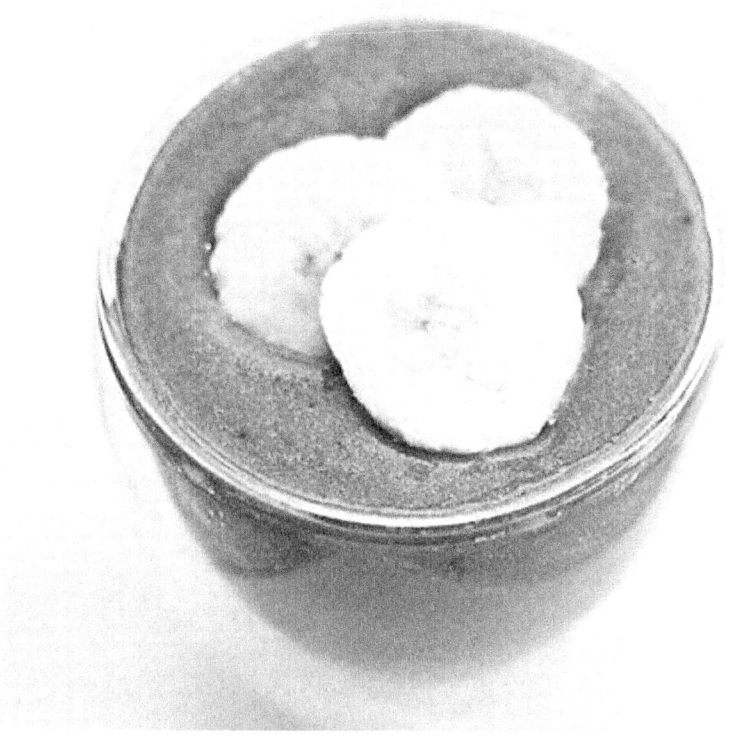

Ingredients

Banana: 1

Peaches: 2

Spinach leaves: 2 handfuls

Water: 1 cup

Directions

Take a food processor or blender and pour all the ingredients in it. Process them until smooth. Add more water if desirable. Spinach-kiwi green smoothie is ready to drink.

Spinach Smoothie with Watermelon and Strawberries

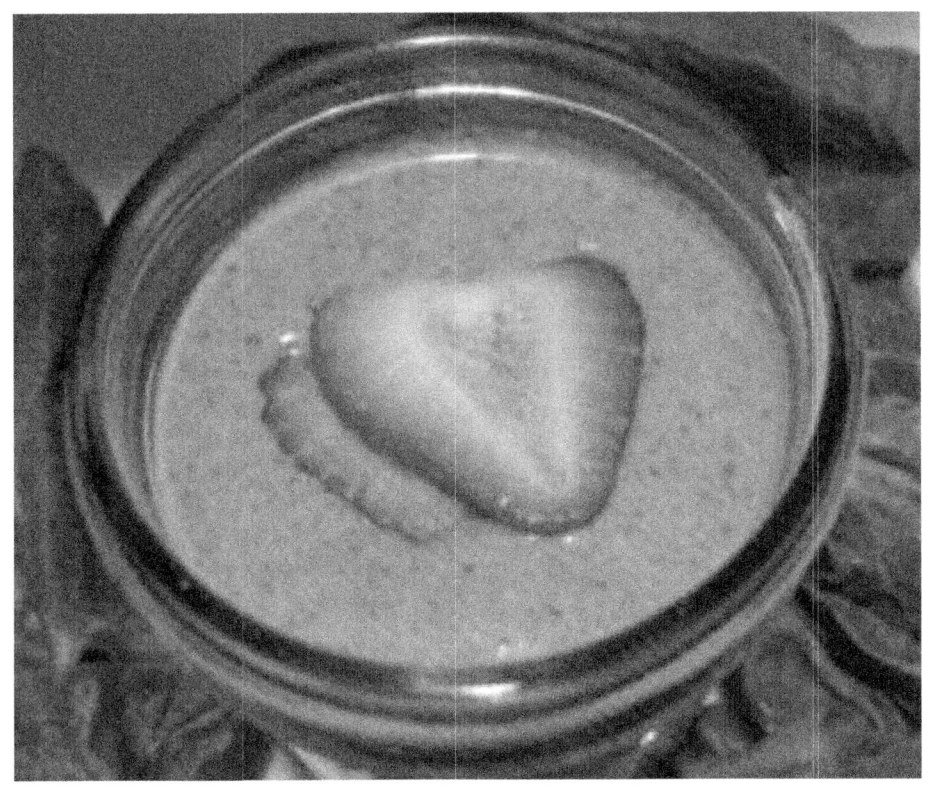

Ingredients

Watermelon (peeled and seeded): 1 half piece

Strawberries: 10

Spinach: 1 bunch

Water: 1 cup

Directions

Take a food processor or blender and pour all the ingredients in it. Process them until smooth. Add more water if desirable. Spinach Smoothie with Watermelon and Strawberries is ready to drink.

Orange Smoothie with Spinach and Banana

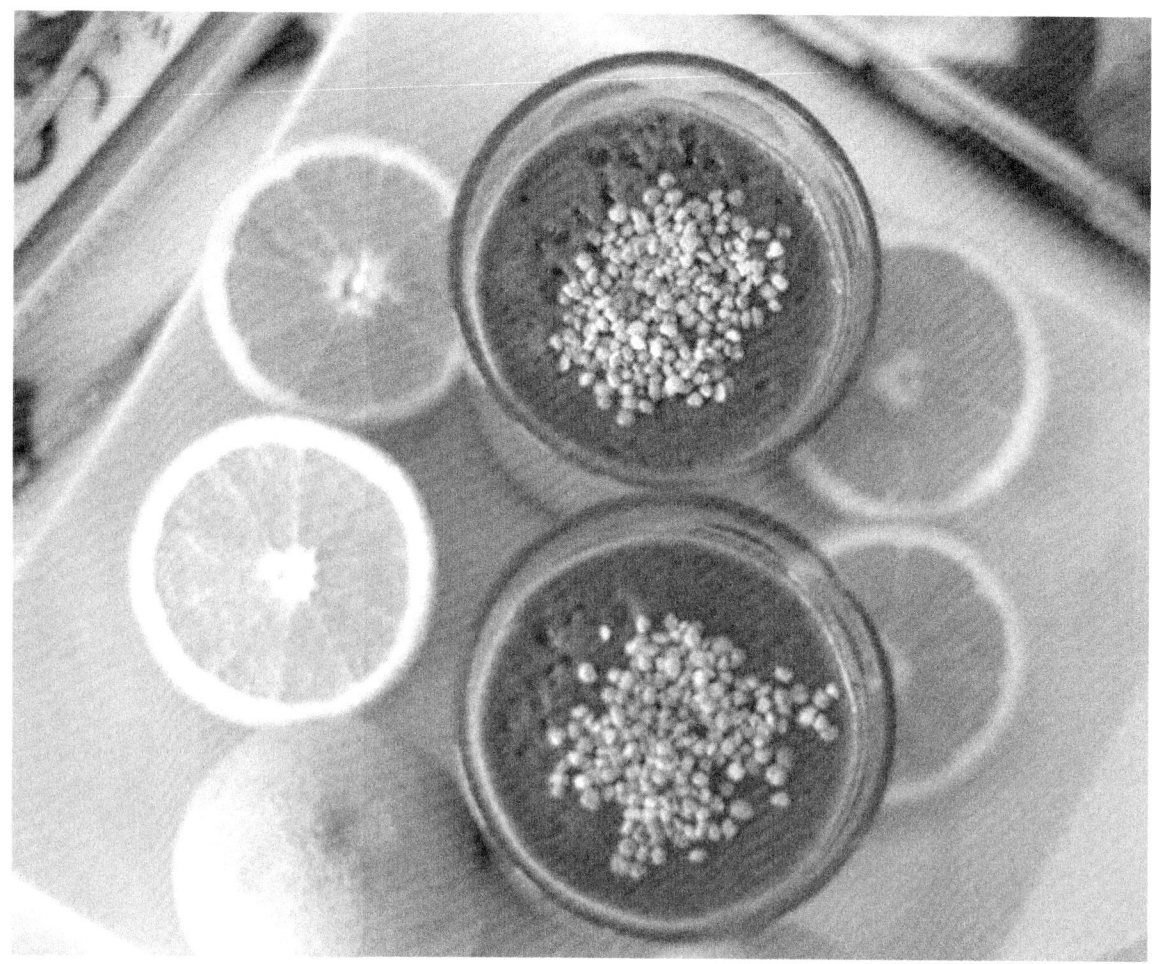

Ingredients

Ripe bananas (large): 2

Oranges: 2

Baby spinach: 2 handfuls

Directions

Take a food processor or blender and pour all the ingredients in it. Process them until smooth. Add more water if desirable. Orange Smoothie with Spinach and Bananas ready to drink.

Spinach and Tomato Smoothie

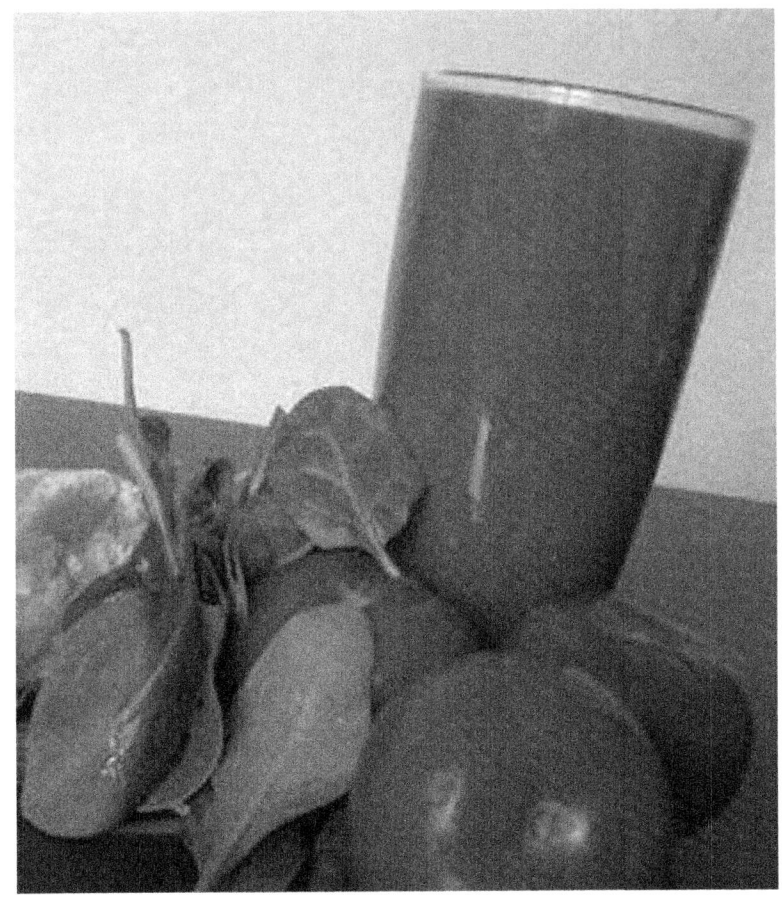

Ingredients

Ripe and plum tomatoes: 4

Spinach leaves: 1 handful

Basil leaves: 4 leaves

Directions

Take a food processor or blender and pour all the ingredients in it. Process them until smooth. Add more water if desirable. Spinach And Tomato Smoothie is ready to drink.

Green Limeade Smoothie

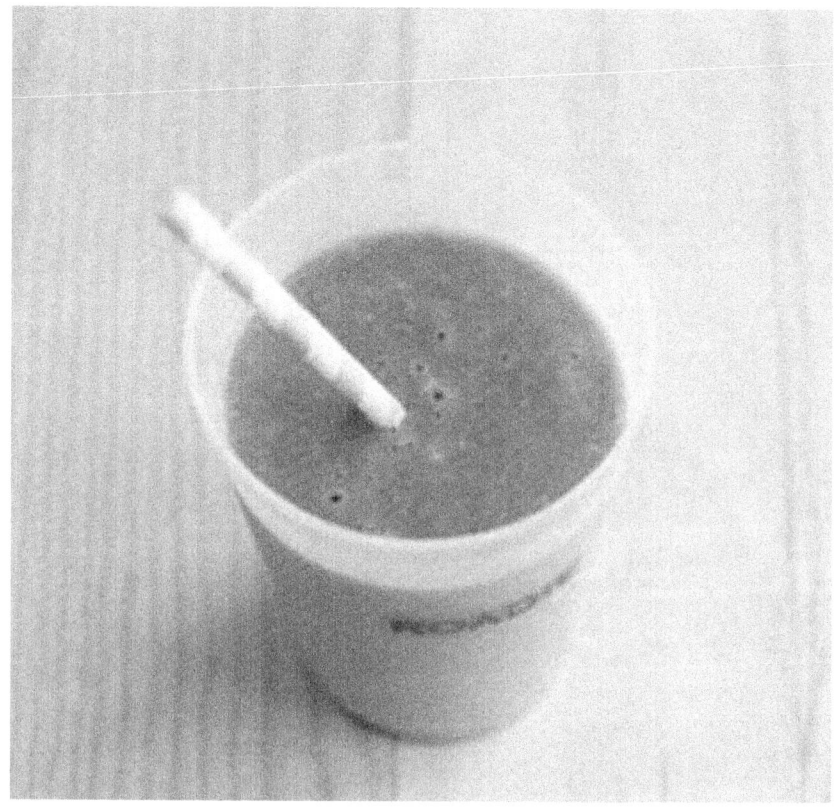

Ingredients

English cucumber (sliced): ½

Avocado: ½

Baby spinach: 2 handfuls

Limes (peeled): 3 to 4

Cinnamon: ½ teaspoon

Honey: According to taste

Ice cubes: 6 to 8

Directions

Take a food processor or blender and put all the ingredients in it. Process them until smooth. Add more water if desirable. Green Limeade Smoothie is ready to drink.

Grapes Smoothie

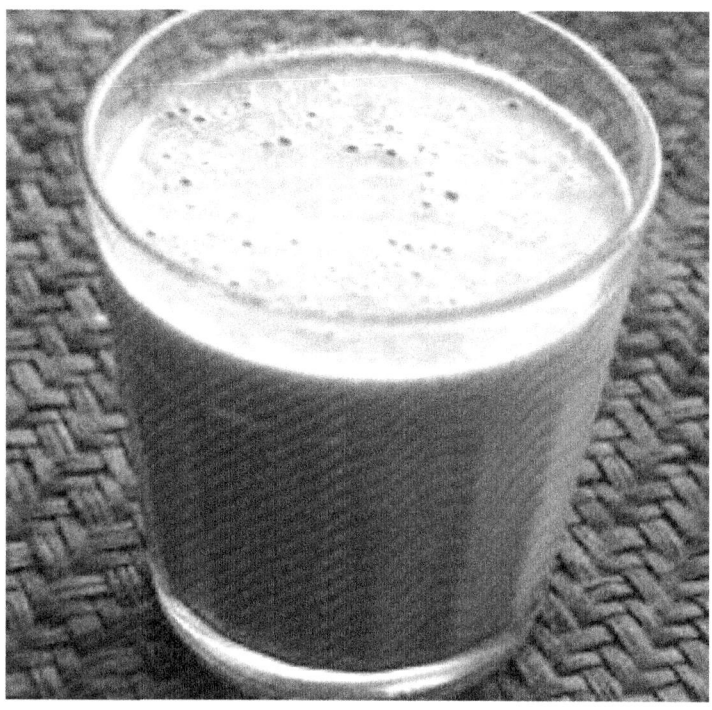

Ingredients

Banana (cut into chunks): 1

Grapes: 1 cup

Low-fat vanilla yogurt: 6 ounce

Apple (cored, chopped): ½

Fresh spinach: 1 ½ cups

Directions

Take a food processor or blender and put all the ingredients in it. Process them until smooth. Stop frequently to ensure that any of the ingredients does not stuck in the blender. Add more water if desirable. Pour into the glass. Grapes Smoothie is ready to drink.

Kale Smoothie

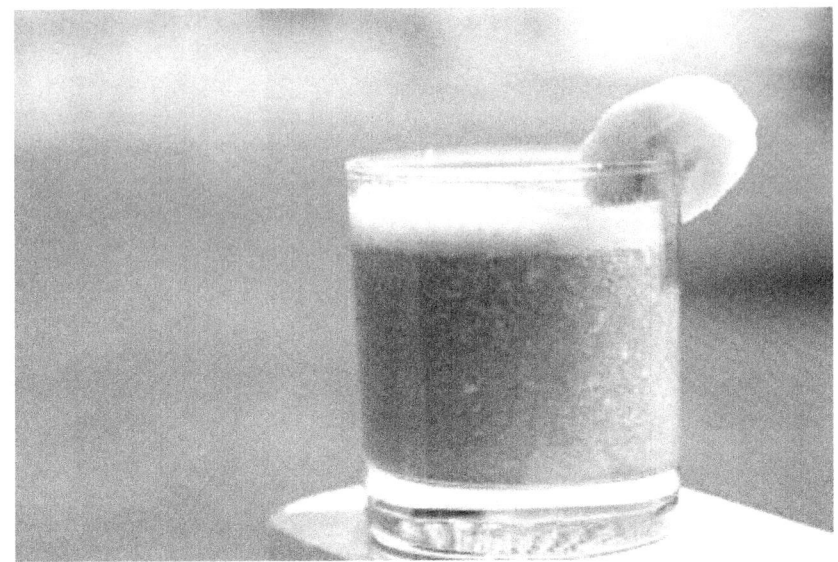

Ingredients

Banana: 1

Chopped kale: 2 cups

Soy milk (light and unsweetened): ½ cup

Flax seeds: 1 tablespoon

Maple syrup: 1 teaspoon

Directions

Take a food processor or blender and put all the ingredients in it. Process them until smooth. Add more water if desirable. Kale Smoothie is ready to drink.

Avocado Smoothie

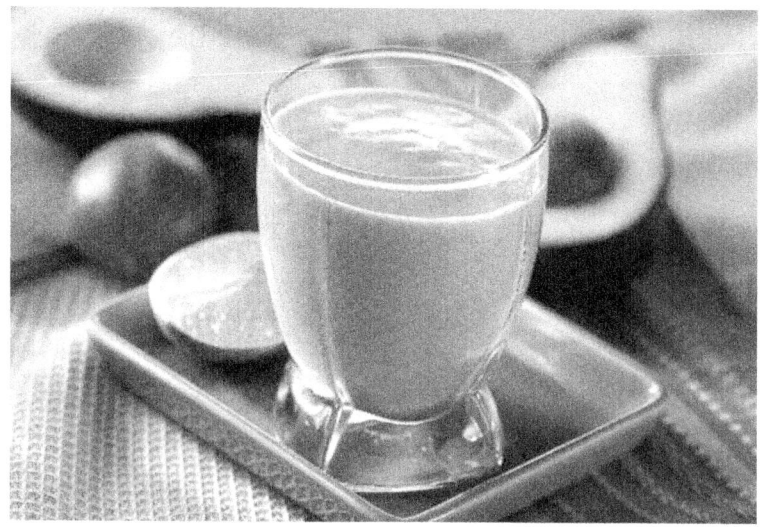

Ingredients

Ripe avocado (halved, pitted): 1

Low-fat milk: 1 cup

Low-fat vanilla yogurt: ½ cup

Honey: 3 tablespoons

Ice cubes: 8

Directions

Take a food processor and put all the ingredients in it. Process them until smooth. Add more water if desirable. Avocado smoothie is ready to drink.

Honeydew Melon Smoothie

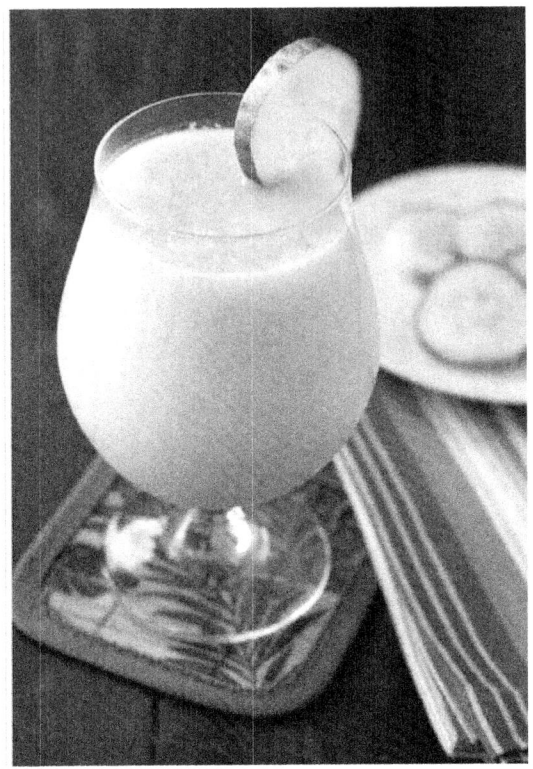

Ingredients

Honeydew melon (peeled, seeded, cubed): 3 cups

Ice cubes: 3 cups

Green grapes: 1 cup

Cucumber (peeled, chopped): 1

Broccoli florets: ½ cup (optional)

Fresh mint: 1 sprig

Directions

Take a food processor or blender and pour all the ingredients in it. Process them until smooth. Add more water if desirable. Honeydew Melon Smoothie is ready to drink.

Ginger and Spinach Smoothie

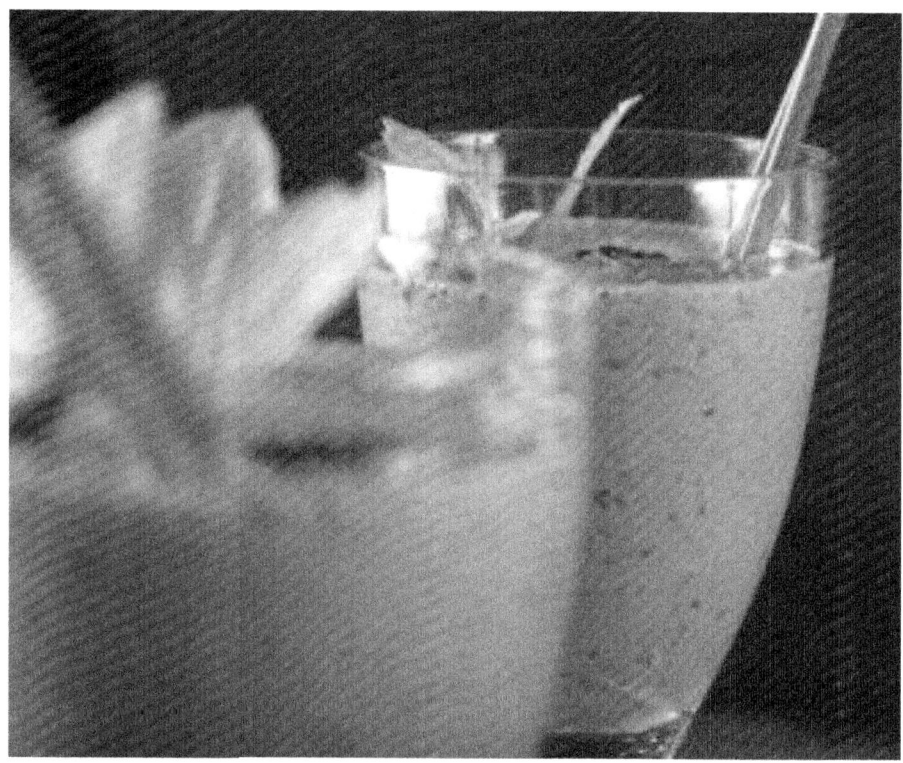

Ingredients

Organic blueberries (frozen): 1 cup

Fresh spinach: 2 cups

Water: 2 cups

Ginger root: ½ inch or according to taste

Directions

Take a food processor or blender and pour all the ingredients in it. Process them until smooth. Add more water if desirable. Ginger and Spinach Smoothie is ready to drink.

Green Coconut Smoothie with Spinach

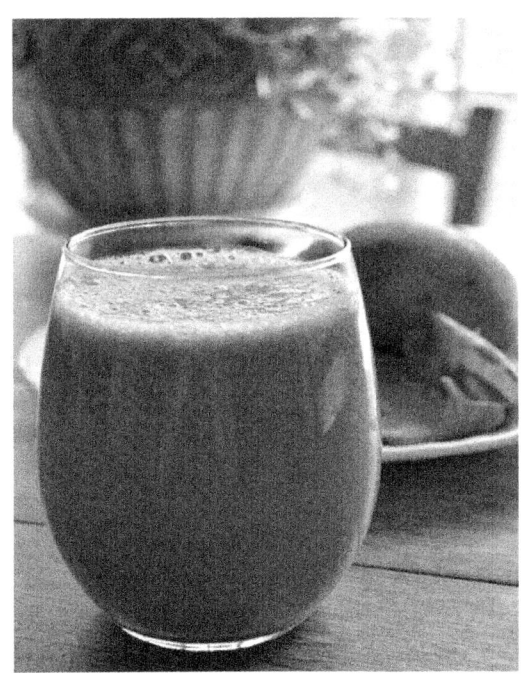

Ingredients

Frozen bananas: 2

Spinach: 2 handfuls

Low-fat almond milk: 1 cup

Cinnamon: ¼ teaspoon

Vanilla: 1 teaspoon

Coconut oil: 1 tablespoon

Directions

Take a food processor or blender and pour all the ingredients in it. Process them until smooth. Add more water if desirable. Pour the smoothie into the glass. Green Coconut Smoothie with Spinach is ready to drink.

Green Apple and Cinnamon Smoothie

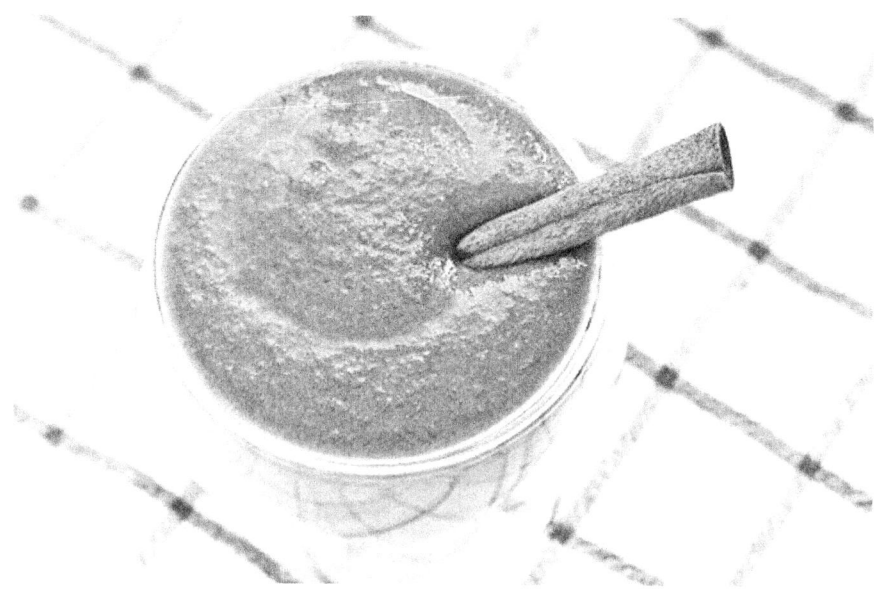

Ingredients

Apple juice: 1 cup

Pear (cored, sliced): 1

Apple (cored, sliced): 1

Fresh spinach: 1 cup

Ground cinnamon: 1 teaspoon

Ice: ½ cup

Directions

Take a food processor or blender and pour all the ingredients in it. Process them until smooth. Add more water if desirable. Green Apple and Cinnamon Smoothie is ready to drink.

Low-Fat Honey and Green Tea Smoothie

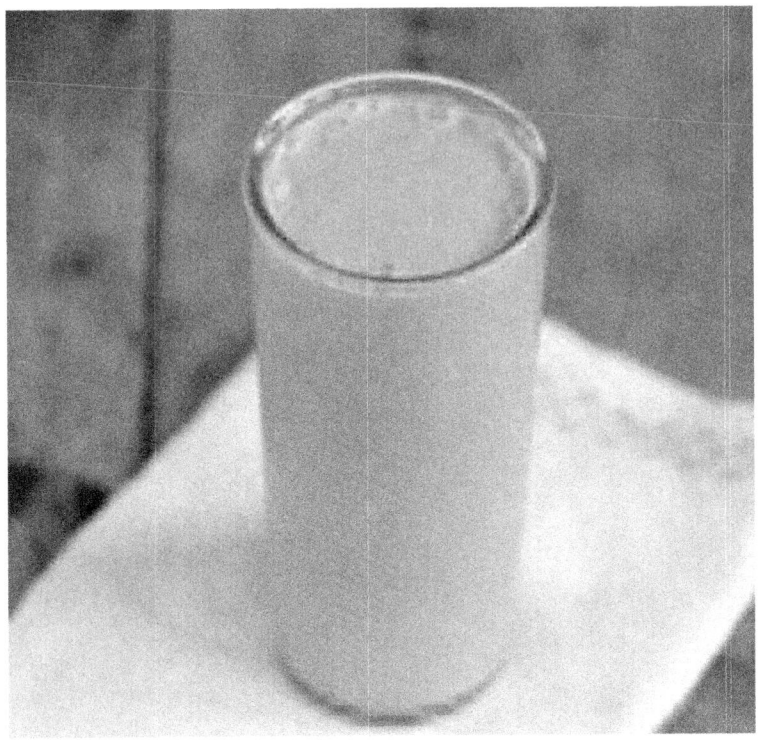

Ingredients

Low-fat frozen yogurt (vanilla): ½ cup

Green tea (chilled): ¼ cup

Honey: 1 tablespoon

Ice: 1 cup

Ground nutmeg

Ground cinnamon

Directions

Take a food processor or blender and pour all the ingredients in it. Process them until smooth. Add more water if desirable. Low-Fat Honey and Green Tea Smoothie is ready to drink.

Dandelion Green Smoothie

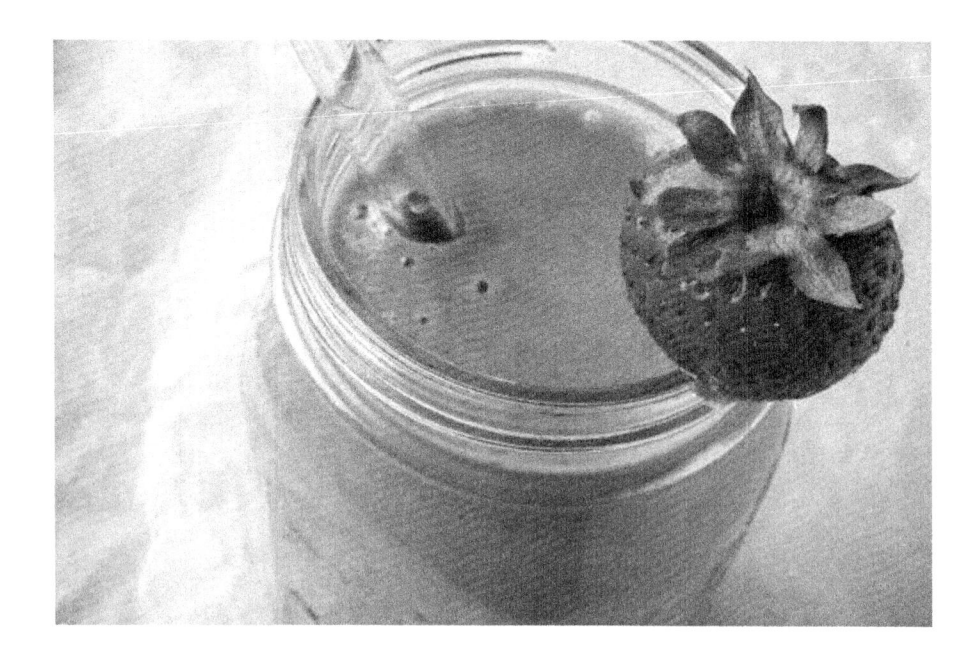

Ingredients

Dandelion greens: 3 cups

Apple juice: 2 cups

Water: 1 cup

Mango: 1

Peach: 1

Directions

Take a food processor or blender and pour all the ingredients in it. Process them until smooth. Add more water if desirable. Dandelion Green Smoothie is ready to drink.

Green Fruity Smoothie

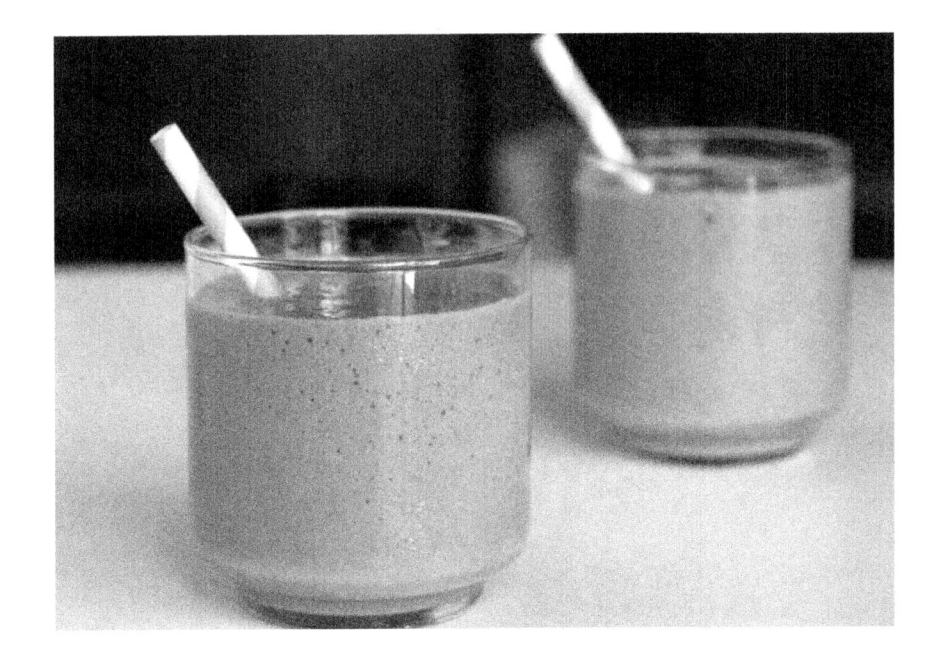

Ingredients

Cored apple: 1

Packed spinach: 2 cups

Greek yogurt: ½ cup

Orange juice: 1/3 cup

Oranges: 1 ½

Flax seed (ground): 2 tablespoons

Honey: ½ tablespoon

Pineapple juice: 6 oz

Banana (frozen): 1

Ice: 1 ½ cups

Directions

1. Take a food processor or blender and pour all the ingredients in it. Process them until smooth. Add more water if desirable.

2. Take out 2 glasses, and pour the smoothie into them. Green Fruity Smoothie is ready to drink.

Mixed Greens Smoothie

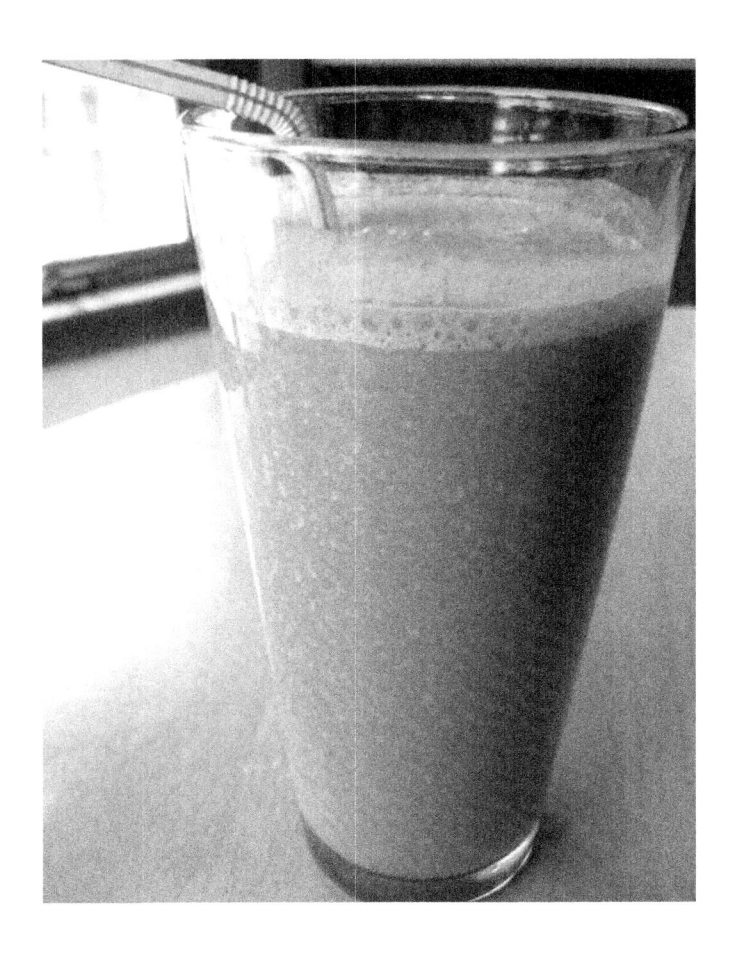

Ingredients

Mixed fruit: 1 ½ cups

Mixed greens: 1 cup

Wheat germ: 1 tablespoon

Low-fat almond milk: 1 cup approx.

Directions

Take a food processor or blender and pour all the ingredients in it. Process them until smooth. Add more water if desirable. Mixed Greens Smoothie is ready to drink.

Collard Green Smoothie

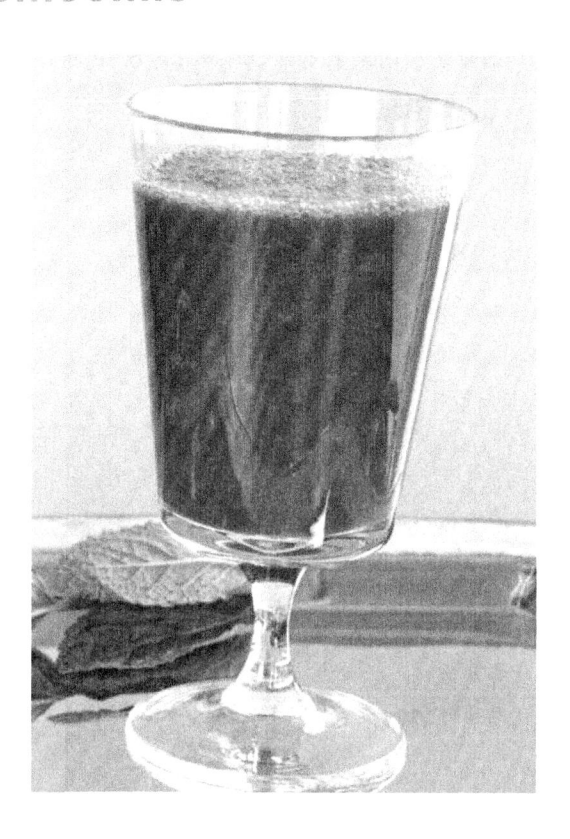

Ingredients

Ripe banana (large): 1

Collard greens (packed): 1 ½ cups

Pineapple (canned or fresh): ¾ cup

Kiwi (peeled): 1

Stevia: ¼ to ½ teaspoon

Blueberries (frozen): ¾ cup

Ice cubes: 3

Water: 1 cup

Directions

1. Take a food processor or blender. Place the greens and fresh fruit in the blender first. These ingredients should be close to the blade.

2. Now, add the remaining ingredients. Process them until smooth. Add more water if desirable. Collard Green Smoothie is ready to drink.

Kiwi Smoothie with Berry and Collards

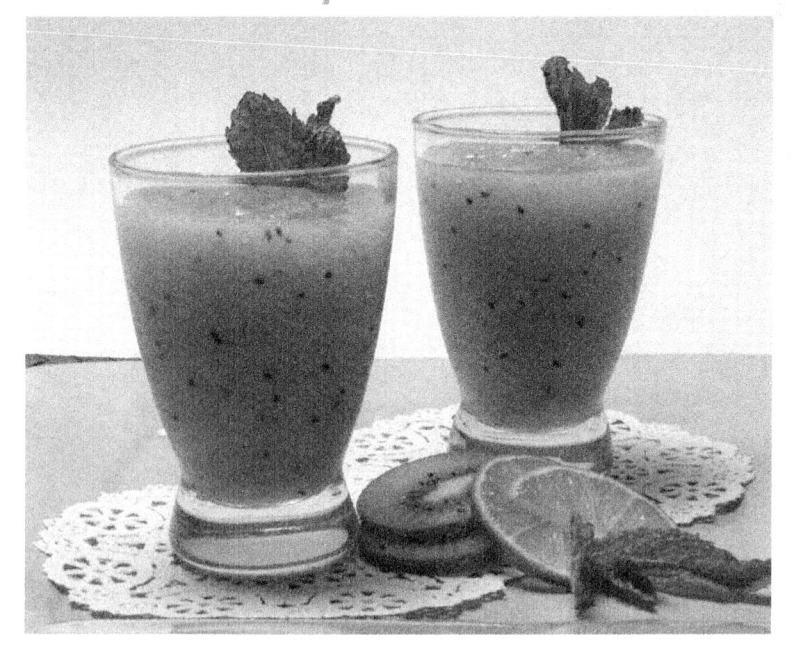

Ingredients

Ripe banana (large): 1

Fresh collard greens: 1 to 2 cups

Kiwi (peeled): 1

Frozen blueberries: ¾ cup

Frozen mangoes: ¾ cup

Stevia: 1 packet

Water: 1 cup

Directions

1. Take a blender, and place the banana in it first. It should be near the blade.

2. Pour the remaining ingredients onto the blender, and blend all the ingredients until they are smooth. Add more water if desirable. Kiwi Smoothie with Berry and Collards is ready to drink.

Fresh Collard Smoothie with Strawberries

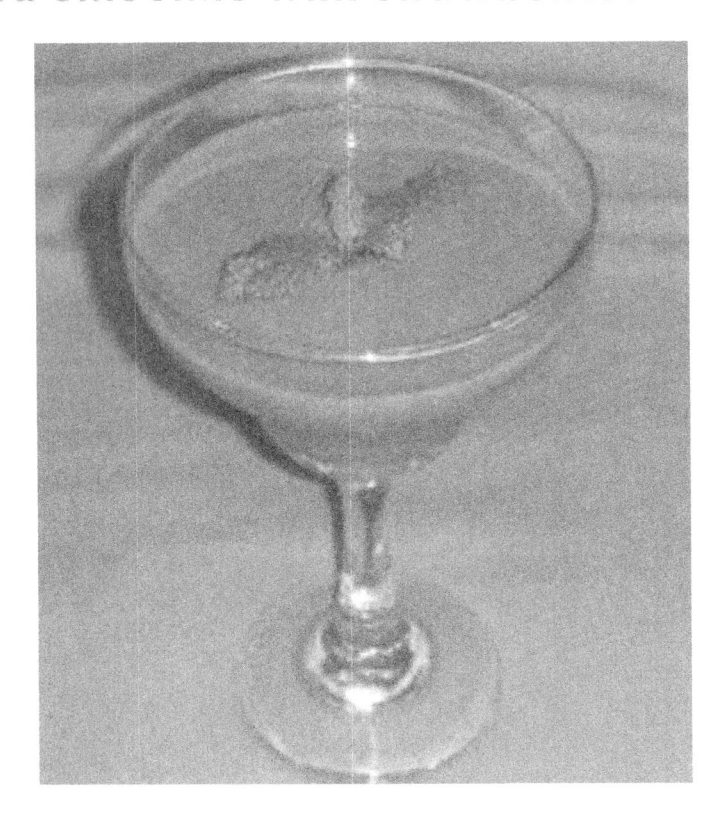

Ingredients

Ripe banana (large): 1

Fresh collard greens: 1 to 2 cups

Fresh strawberries: 1 cup

Frozen mangoes: ¾ cup

Ice cubes: 3

Stevia: 1 packet

Water: 1 ½ cups

Directions

1. Take a blender, and place the banana in it first. It should be near the blade.

2. Pour the remaining ingredients onto the blender, and blend all the ingredients until they are smooth. Add more water if desirable. Fresh Collard Smoothie with Strawberries is ready to drink.

Final Word

Now that you have learnt what it takes to prepare a delicious and fat burning smoothie from different green fruits and vegetables, you can have a glass of your favorite smoothie anytime of the day.

Whether you want to start your day with kiwi fruit smoothie or add a bit of strawberries and collard greens in it, you will be able to get rid of those extra pounds while a glass of drinking nutritious and fat-burning smoothie. If your family and friends want to achieve the same weight-loss goal as yours, then sharing another glass of green smoothie is the best you can give them!

Printed in Great Britain
by Amazon